ALBIE

The Bipolar Bear

BY

JAMIE BENNETT

ILLUSTRATED BY TIM DUMAS

EDITED BY

KAREN SUE REDLACK

Piranha Publishing

DEDICATIONS

This book is dedicated to all of those that silence themselves and don't want to speak of their time in a hospital for fear of indifference and judgement when it comes to mental health. To all the amazing individuals who work and dedicate their lives to help the healing and understanding of the mind and all its emotions. To those who love and walk along side of us and our journey with mental illness that bring us acceptance and a sense of belonging. To God for giving us feelings so that we can experience those special moments in life that make a smile or a tear.

TABLE OF CONTENTS

INTRODUCTION

Mental illness has been a very big part of my life resulting in several hospitalizations and numerous medications. The lessons, things I have learned and people I've met, have influenced me in my journey. Some of the most memorable are from hospitals. I decided on writing this book eight years ago while attending a Partial Hospitalization Program (PHP) at Cedar Ridge Behavioral Center, a psychiatric hospital. I was there for my Bipolar Disorder. PHP was to teach us how to regain our confidence to go back to our lives after our mental health crisis.

The name Albie came from another patient with Dementia and Bipolar. I wanted to tell a story to bring enlightenment to mental health and times spent in hospitals where the stay isn't always pleasant. Still, it shouldn't be frowned upon or make the person feel any less than wonderfully created. Hospitalization is sometimes a taboo subject. I want Albie and his friends to make it an adventure with fun times, relatable feelings and emotions. It is always better to seek assistance when facing any health issues or concerns. It takes great strength to admit when we need help and securing that help can make a positive difference for all of us.

ACKNOWLEDGMENTS

Thank you to my Mother for her undying love, never giving up hope on me with the countless trips to hospitals, doctor visits and medication trials. I love ya nag! To my Father for always having a prayer for me.

Thank you to my two amazing children, Maddi and Nate, who have given me inspiration and encouragement to press forward and find true joy in my life.

Thanks to my extended family and friends for always providing safe spaces for me with understanding and love.

Thank you to my workplace family, Uptown Grocery, for giving me support and inclusion with my mental health.

Last, but not least, thank you to Ginny Curtis, the woman whose faith in God led me to the journey of publishing these books.

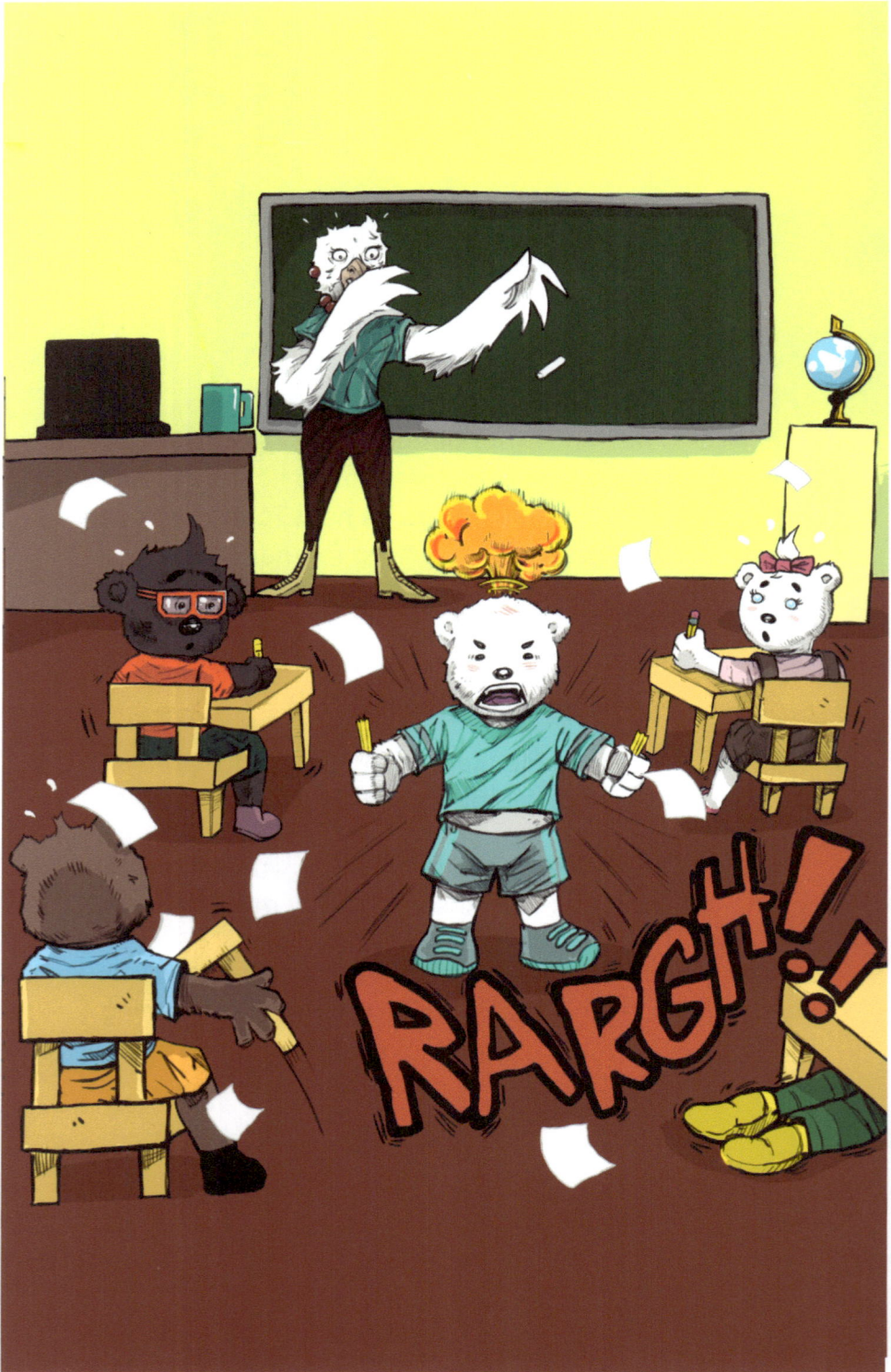

STOMPING, GROWLING AND SNARLING

It was a beautiful morning at Neko Harbour Elementary. Albie, a ten year old polar bear, sat down waiting for Mrs. Albatross to start her lesson. All the other classmates were waiting too. Albie started to think about what he would learn today. Albie wanted to be an explorer. He loved to travel to different places with his dad. They had been all over Antarctica. Albie had seen so many amazing places. He met all kinds of interesting animals and tasted delicious foods as well.

Mrs. Albatross came into the room and rang the bell to let everyone know class was about to begin. The students got quiet and Mrs. Albatross announced that today they would be learning about geography. OH MY, Albie thought. This was so exciting! Geography was his favorite subject. Mrs. Albatross asked if anyone knew the location of Mount Erebus. Albie knew this immediately. Mount Erebus was a volcano and it was on Ross Island! He raised his paw as fast and high as he could! PICK ME! PICK ME! Albie thought to himself. Mrs. Albatross decided to ask another student, Shayla! OH NO! Albie thought, I wanted to answer that. He got so angry! That wasn't fair! He loved geography and knew that answer. Albie started to GROWL AND SNARL! He couldn't help it. He

11

started stomping his paws! He was so angry because he didn't get picked!

Other students started staring at him and he got embarrassed, which only made him sad too. Mrs. Albatross came over to speak to Albie, but he didn't want to talk. He wanted to cry. He didn't understand why he had all this anger and sadness he couldn't control. Mrs. Albatross asked Albie to come outside with her and that hurt him worse! Everyone knew something was wrong and he still couldn't control it.

Albie went outside to the hallway with Mrs. Albatross. She asked if he wanted to call his Mom. Albie told her with another growl, "No, I wanted to answer the question! I know the answer, but you picked Shayla," he screamed. "I just want to answer the question!" He growled and stomped.

While whistling with a smile on his face, around the corner came one of Albie's dearest friends, Counselor Prion. He could see Albie was upset. Counselor Prion was a very wise bird. Students at Neko Harbour Elementary could talk to him about anything and he was always very helpful. He knew Albie and his family long before Albie was born. He had served in the Arctic military with Albie's Dad, Colonel Polar Bear. When Counselor Prion and Colonel Polar Bear got together they always had cool stories to tell.

As soon as Albie saw Counselor Prion he forgot why he was so upset and started smiling. He gave Counselor Prion a big hug and asked if he could go with him to his office to look at all his maps and pictures. Counselor Prion had maps and pictures of all the different places he had been. Mrs. Albatross agreed to let Albie go with him and she went back to her classroom.

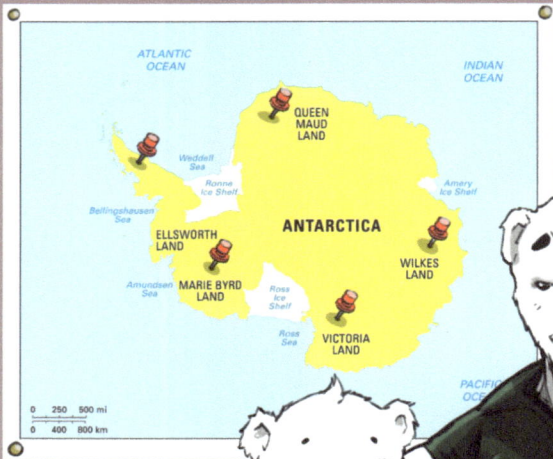

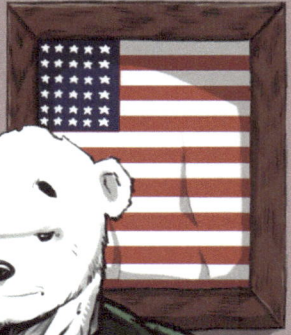

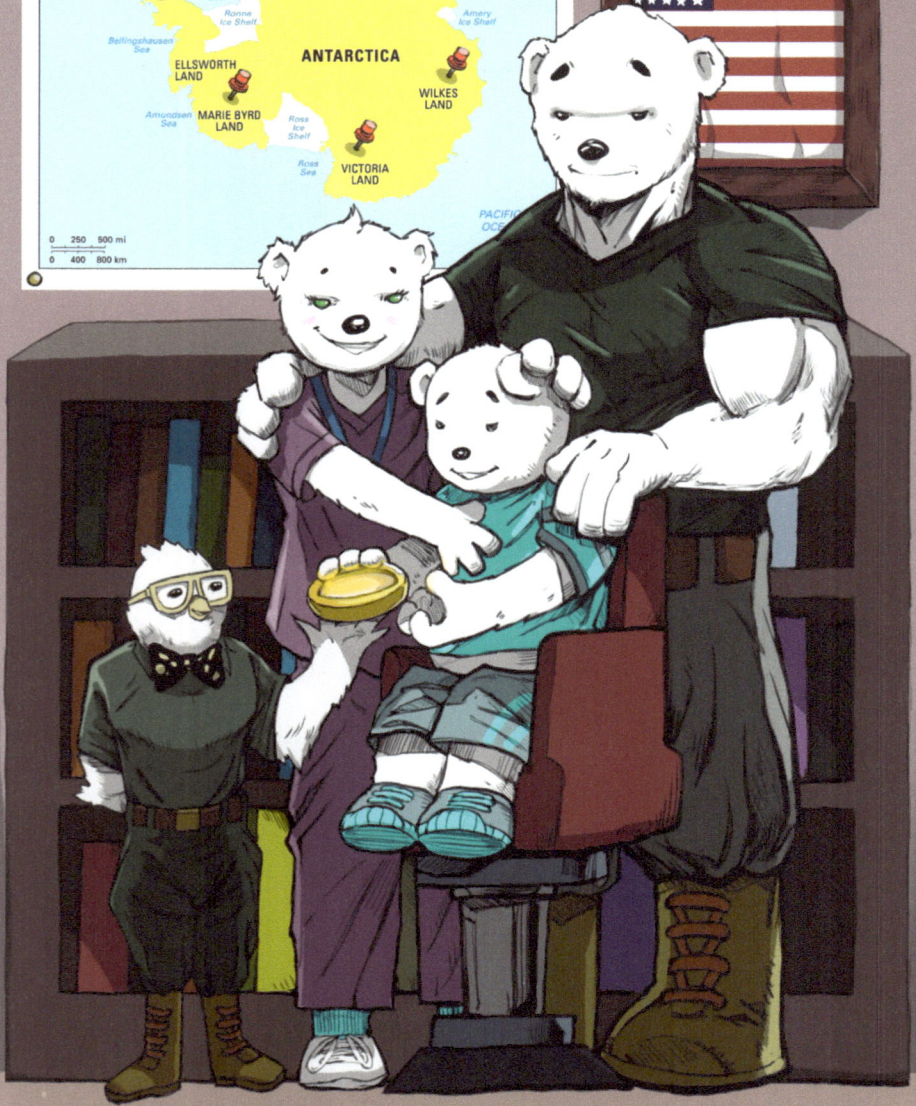

A COMPASS FOR ALBIE'S ADVENTURES

Counselor Prion gave Albie a map of all the places he had been to in Antarctica. It was marked with special colors where he had visited. Some were for fun and others for his time in the service. He saw that Albie was calming down and decided to ask him what happened to get him so upset. Albie told him he couldn't help but to growl, snarl and stomp. He said he even cried because he didn't get picked to answer the question. Everyone had been watching him so that made him feel worse.

Albie told Counselor Prion he didn't mean to get angry and growl at his classmates and Mrs. Albatross, but he couldn't help it. Counselor Prion explained to Albie that it was okay to get angry, but he just needed to learn how to control the way he reacted to his anger without growling, snarling and stomping. Albie agreed and once again looked at the map. Albie told Counselor Prion he wanted to be a great explorer and go all over Antarctica and the world.

He was having so many pictures in his mind and his thoughts were going so fast. Albie looked at the map and began to say "I want to go here, here and there!" He started thinking about geography again and the question in class. He started to get upset. Counselor Prion could see Albie was having some troubles again so he decided to call his parents. Albie thought he might be in trouble, but Counselor Prion assured him it was only to help him. His Mom and Dad would want to know if he was having a hard day. Besides, he said it would give him and Albie's Dad a chance to catch up on old military stories. Albie's mother and father loved him very much. His Dad and Albie would go exploring and fishing and his Mom always made his favorite sushi! Albie's Mom was a nurse at Neko Harbour Hospital and his Dad worked down at the shipyard. Albie loved his parents very much as well so he was excited to see them when they came into Counselor Prion's office. He ran up and gave them both a huge hug.

Albie was so happy everyone was there he forgot all about his anger and crying. Now he just wanted to sit and visit and show them the map of Antarctica that he had. Albie looked down at the map while his parents and Counselor Prion talked. He saw Mount Erebus marked on the map and remembered why he was there in the first place. He began to get upset again. Albie started crying and he got really sad. He remembered everyone noticed his anger. What would they think of him now? Counselor Prion looked at Albie and told him he had something very special for him. He opened a drawer and pulled out a shiny round object and a map. Counselor Prion told Albie that the shiny round thing was called a compass and it would always help him go in the right direction. Counselor Prion said, "All great explorers have compasses, Albie."

"Wow!" said Albie, "This is amazing! I really am an explorer now." HIs tears dried and a smile came through. Counselor Prion then explained to Albie and his parents that the map was of a wonderful place with a very special doctor. It was Neko Harbour Mental Health Hospital. Counselor Prion knew Albie could get the help he needed there.

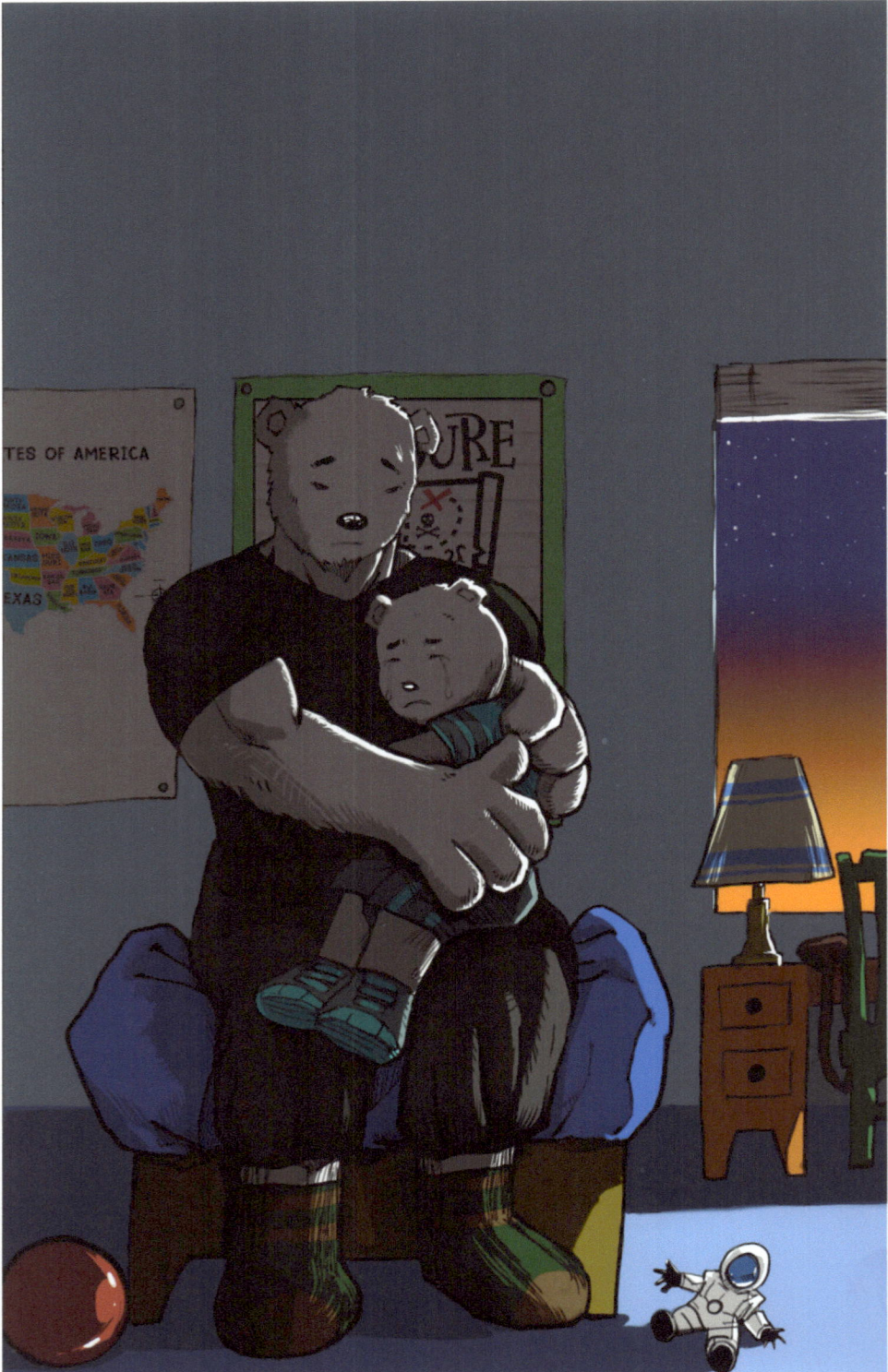

A FATHER'S LOVE AND SUPPORT FOR A NEW PLACE

Albie and his parents waited in Counselor Prion's office while he called and set up an appointment for the following day. Albie was to meet with Dr. Nori. She was a well known psychiatrist that worked at the hospital. Counselor Prion was Dr. Nori's very dear friend. He knew she was just the Orca for Albie to talk to. She had traveled all the way from Cape Reynard by the Onyx River. Dr. Nori was a killer whale, the largest Orca around and very well trained in her field of study which was psychiatry. Counselor Prion trusted her to help Albie with his episode.

Albie and his parents said goodbye to Counselor Prion and headed home. They were all hungry so Albie's Mom made some sushi and then it was time for bed. Albie was wide awake looking at the compass and hospital map. There were so many neat places on the map of the hospital. Albie started wondering what Dr. Nori would be like and what they would talk about. Albie opened his compass and looked at the North Star. It was right above his bedroom window and the moonlight lit up Neko Harbour. Albie closed his eyes and fell fast asleep right by the window.

Albie had so many questions for Dr. Nori the day of the visit. He was excited to meet a new doctor. Albie's Mom was a nurse at Neko Harbour. He had been to visit her there many times. Albie's Mom explained to him that Dr. Nori was a different kind of doctor than what she worked with. Dr. Nori was a psychiatrist and she would help Albie with his mental health.

His Mom explained the difference between mental health and physical health. Mental was the mind and physical was the body. Albie didn't understand. His mind wasn't hurting. He knew nothing was broken so why go to a hospital or doctor? He started getting confused with things and scared about the hospital. He didn't think anything was wrong with him. He wasn't happy or excited now. In fact, he wasn't sure if he even wanted to go to the doctor now. Why would they want him to if he wasn't sick? Albie got upset then and the closer it got the less excited he became. Albie's Mom knew this was a job for someone very special to Albie. Albie needed someone who was courageous and brave. They needed to know about being scared and talking to a psychiatrist. Albie's Dad, Colonel Polar Bear had served in the Arctic Army and after his service he had to visit a well known psychiatrist at Onyx River many times.

Albie's Dad went to his son's room and sat next to him. He hugged him tight. He could see Albie was scared. Albie loved his Father's hugs. They started talking about all the times that his Dad had been away in the military and how brave he had been. Albie listened to his Dad while he told him something Albie never knew. Colonel Polar Bear had also visited a mental health hospital and seen The Great Blue Whale Dr.

Dash, a psychiatrist. Albie had no idea his Dad was ever sick and even went to the hospital!

Colonel Polar Bear assured his son that they were going to get this all figured out about what happened to Albie at school and all would be fine. He said, "Albie you are going to have to be brave. This will be a new adventure." Albie could explore all the hospitals as they helped him. Albie got his compass, map and put them into his satchel and told his Dad he was ready to go.

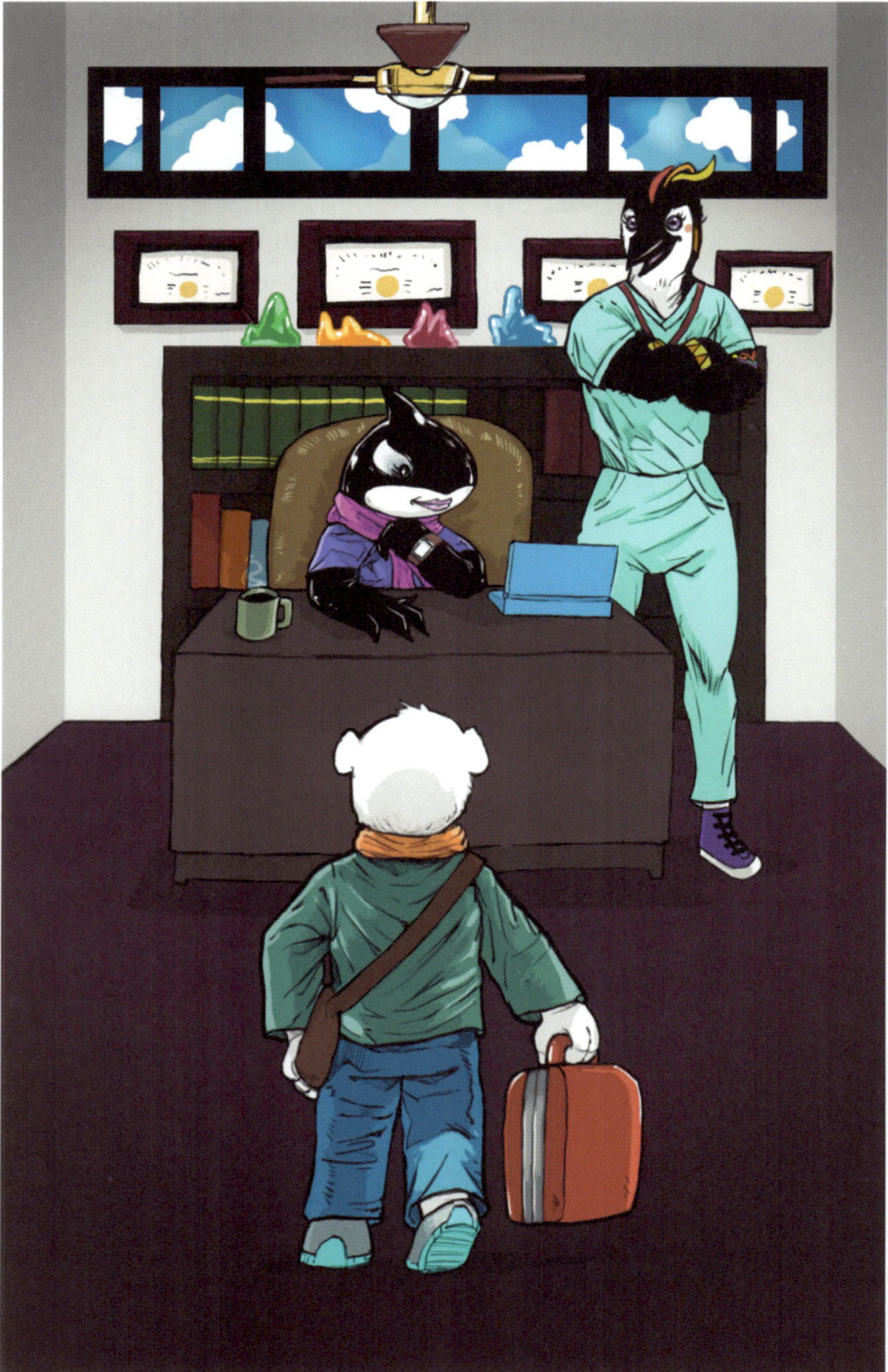

NEKO HARBOUR'S
MENTAL HEALTH HOSPITAL

Albie and his parents got to Neko Harbour Hospital and went to an area that was new to Albie. It wasn't like the part where his mother worked. There were no bandages or people coughing. Nobody sounded sick there. Some looked happy, some looked sad and some were just talking amongst themselves. The hospital sounded kind of fun. Albie could hear music coming from one area.

They went up to the front desk and he met a very colorful Emperor Penguin with rainbow tattoos all over her neck and chest. She had a big smile on her face. With a cheerful voice she said, "Hello, I am Artemis, a nurse here at Neko Harbour!" Albie quickly responded with an excited, "Hello, I'm Albie!" Mrs. Polar Bear told Artemis they were there to see Dr. Nori.

Artemis opened the door for them and Albie saw a long hallway full of windows. He started to get a little nervous and grabbed his Father's paw. Colonel Polar Bear looked at his son and reminded him to be brave. Artemis complimented Albie's satchel. Albie said, "Thank you. It has my maps and compass in it." OH YEAH! His maps and compass! Why didn't he think of that? Every explorer needed their map and compass.

Albie stopped right then and there and got them out of his satchel. "Look," he showed Artemis. "This is a map of the hospital and here is my compass. We are going north." Artemis looked at the compass. "Is this some kind of magic? I have never seen a compass before." Albie told her what it was used for and that Counselor Prion gave it to him. Then he showed her the map of the hospital and she pointed to a place and said, "This is where we are going!" with a big smile.

Artemis made Albie feel very comfortable and she didn't scare him at all. She hummed and sang songs to herself as they walked through the hospital. They came up to one room and she told Albie, "If you ever feel sad or unhappy you can go in this room and listen to music or dance! Either way it's a wonderful way to heal your mind." Albie would remember that he liked music a lot. He looked on his map and saw a room that said Art and asked Artemis about it.

She smiled again and led them down another hallway where they came up to a purple door covered in yellow and green flowers. It said ART in big letters. Artemis opened the door and it was awesome! There were paints, coloring books, easels and all different colored pencils. There were also beads to make jewelry with so many neat and wonderful things to do in there. As much as Albie's parents were enjoying the tour it was almost time for Albie's appointment with Dr. Nori. She told Albie that the Art room was always open and he would have to come back and visit it.

Artemis took the family to the second floor of the hospital to a couple of sliding glass doors. "This is Dr. Nori's office," she said. "She is waiting for you." Colonel Polar Bear opened the door. To Albie's surprise his eyes lit up to see Counselor Prion sitting in a chair. He had no idea he was going to be there! Albie hugged him and turned around to see a very majestic creature! She had blue eyes. She was very tall and with a pleasant voice said, "Hello, I am Dr. Nori." Albie couldn't speak for a moment. Dr. Nori was so magnificent. He had never seen a killer whale before. Albie was so intrigued by the Orca he almost forgot where he was.

Albie's Mother and Father said, "Hello." Albie finally said hello as well. Dr. Nori had all kinds of certifications on her walls and a shelf with what looked like crystals and gemstones. She and Albie's parents were sitting and talking. Counselor Prion sat and listened while Albie started to get a little anxious again. He held onto his compass tight. Someone called out his name, "Albie?" Dr. Nori said. "How are you feeling today? Are you sad, mad or happy?" Albie told her he was feeling scared earlier because he didn't feel sick and couldn't understand why he had to come to the hospital. He continued to tell her he was excited to see Counselor Prion and to meet Dr. Nori, but was still confused.

Dr. Nori asked Albie if he remembered how he felt at school the day before. Albie thought about what happened. He began to look around the room at Counselor Prion and his parents. He was getting a little nervous again. Was he in trouble? Counselor Prion told Albie everything was okay and Dr. Nori was there to help him. Albie opened up and told Dr. Nori about what happened the day before when he had become so mad and sad because he didn't get picked to answer the question. Then he told her he couldn't control his anger so he was growling, snarling and stomping his feet. He told Dr. Nori when he was in Counselor Prion's office he couldn't stop thinking and everything was going fast. He became scared because he didn't know what was wrong with him.

Dr. Nori thanked Albie for trusting her and sharing his story from the day before. She told Albie and his parents she could help him. Dr. Nori wanted him to stay a few days at the hospital so she could watch his sleep patterns and study more of his behaviors. Albie wondered what she meant by behaviors. What was that? He tugged at his Mom's arm and asked her. Dr. Nori overheard and apologized for not explaining things so Albie could understand. She needed to see how he acted around certain situations and others.

She also wanted him to meet a few more of the staff there like he had met Artemis. Albie started to get excited then. Artemis was so nice and made him smile. Albie looked at his parents and agreed to stay there. He didn't know what was going to happen, but he knew he wanted someone to help him. Albie didn't like to be out of control like he had been at school. Dr. Nori assured him he would feel much better after his stay at the hospital. She told Albie and his parents she would like to show them another part of the hospital. Patients just like Albie were there to heal and learn more about their own mental health.

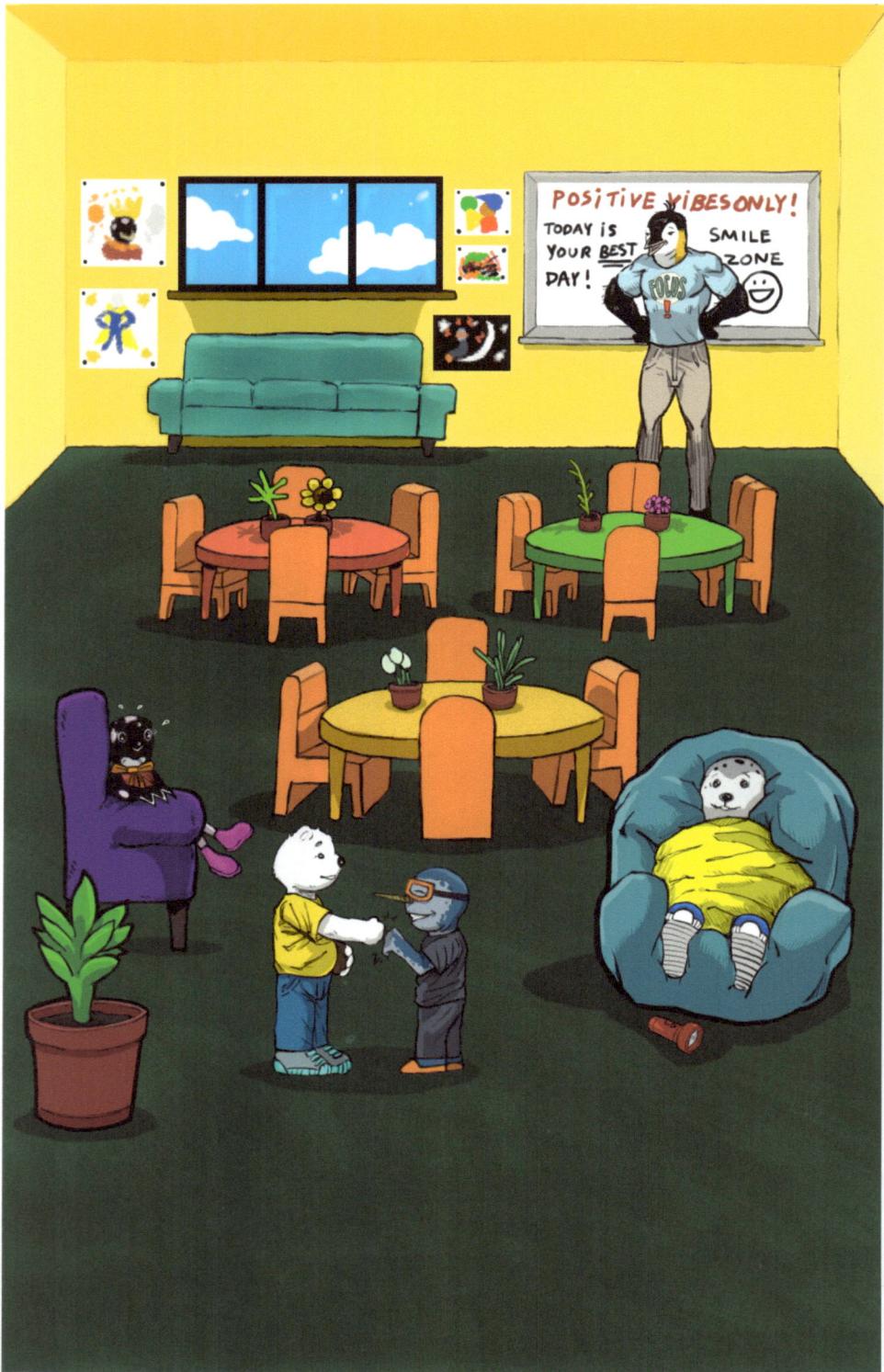

GROUP THERAPY AND NEW FRIENDS

Albie wasn't scared anymore. He was curious what he would find out about himself and his mental health. This was going to be an adventure. A really big one and Albie was the explorer. Counselor Prion had to say goodbye now. He had to go back to school. Albie gave him a big hug. Counselor Prion reminded him of his map and compass. They were tools to help him find his way. He told Albie if he needed him all he had to do was call and he would be right there. Dr. Nori asked Albie and his family to walk with her. Albie quickly grabbed his compass and map then followed.

"I've been to Ross Island before!" "Well I have been to the Polar Ice Caps." Albie heard all these voices while coming down the hall. Dr. Nori led them straight to the doorway and asked Albie if he would like to go sit and join the group with the other patients. Albie turned to his Mom and Dad. "Have courage," his Dad said and patted him on the head as his Mother gave him a warm hug and told him how much she loved him. Albie left his parents behind and went to join the group.

He walked in the room and it was covered with pictures other patients had painted and colored. There was a whiteboard on one wall with all kinds of words that Albie didn't quite understand. There were lots of pretty flowers and plants too. "Well hello there!" Walter quickly said to Albie. "Welcome to the group." Walter was a therapist at the hospital. He was an Emperor Penguin like Artemis. Walter was taller and had huge muscles. He was also a bodybuilder. Albie thought that was awesome!

Walter told Albie to get comfortable. Dr.Nori followed Albie to a turquoise couch by the window. The group was like a class, but different. There weren't as many students and they didn't have any desks. There were different colored couches and a big purple chair that had pillows and a bean bag. One of the patients was a Leopard Seal who had his blanket covering his head. He was making funny noises and holding a yellow flashlight while sitting on the bean bag. Another patient sat on the purple chair with her feet hanging off the side while she shuffled her feathers. She was an Adele Penguin. She was missing patches of her feathers, mostly in the places that her beak had plucked out.

Albie asked Dr. Nori their names and she told him Danny was on the bean bag and Tippy was in the chair. About that time with a very loud yawn and a kind voice someone said, "I have been to Canada and my name is Uni!" Wow! Albie thought! That was thousands of miles away. He got excited because his map at home had shown him that.

Albie was enjoying himself in the group with everyone, but he was still concerned about why he was there. Everyone said it was his mental health, but how does he get better? About that time Albie got a tap on the shoulder. It was a young Narwhal. He introduced himself in a very slow, but friendly voice. "Hi, I'm Uni." He had his diving goggles on. Albie told him they were awesome.

Albie didn't know what to say so he started telling Uni about his maps and showed him the compass that Counselor Prion had given him. He then told Uni he wanted to be an explorer when he grew up. Uni thought that was exciting and told Albie he would go with him to explore. Albie started to forget about being upset and then Uni asked Albie something he didn't know how to answer. "Why are you here Albie"? Uni was curious. Albie froze. He didn't know what to say. He didn't want to get mad and yell, but he really couldn't understand why he was there because he thought he was fine.

Dr. Nori overheard Uni and Albie talking and told Uni that there were a few more processes for Albie before they could be sure about his mental health. "I have Narcolepsy and Depression," said Uni. "I am also an orphan. I got separated from my family while we were migrating." Uni told Albie all the places he had been that he remembered and Albie was fascinated. Albie asked Uni what Narcolepsy and Depression were.

"Well," said Uni." I am always tired with Narcolepsy and sometimes I get very sad with Depression and it's hard for me to think of happy things." Albie didn't know what to say. Uni seemed perfectly normal to him. Uni liked exploring and he had been to many places. Plus he didn't seem sad at all.

Suddenly a cute little penguin jumped up next to him and said,

"HELLO! My name is Tippy!" Tippy was a young penguin with ADHD and Anxiety that made it very hard for her to slow down so she would hum. When Tippy's anxiety would act up she would pluck her feathers. She would get scared and it would be hard for her to breathe.

Tippy asked Albie if she could see his compass and wanted to know more about him. Albie didn't know what to say to her either. He got out his compass and showed her how it worked. Dr. Nori noticed all the attention Albie was getting. She was happy he was getting along with all the other children. She knew it could be hard to be new and comfortable at the hospital.

Albie had been around hospitals his whole life. His mom was a nurse. So far this was not that different. In fact it was better. No one was hurt. There were no bandages, bumps or blood. Then all of a sudden something was wrong. Something that Albie had never experienced before. Danny, the young Leopard Seal, started screaming for help! "They won't stop touching me," he cried." They want to hurt me! Someone please help!" Albie looked over, but he didn't see anyone or anything.

Danny was under his blanket kicking and screaming. Dr. Nori, Walter and Artemis all ran over to Danny. Dr. Nori slowly uncovered him and reminded him of who she was and where he was. She told Artemis to get his medicine. Albie was scared now. What was happening? There wasn't anyone touching Danny that he saw. Uni and Tippy explained to Albie, "Danny has something called Schizophrenia and sometimes he sees and hears things we don't." Tippy looked at Albie and said, "It's okay. Everything will be alright. Danny was having an episode."

Albie felt bad because Danny was scared. Dr. Nori gave Danny his medicine while Walter had to hold him. Albie started thinking, is this mental illness? So when he got mad about Shayla answering the question that was his mental illness? He had a lot of questions and was starting to get nervous. Walter took Danny to his room.

Dr. Nori took Albie outside to say goodbye to his parents. Artemis went back to the room with Tippy and Uni. Albie's Mom and Dad hugged him tight and his Mom told him she would come visit every day after work and Albie could call anytime. Colonel Polar Bear picked his son up and gave him a big squeeze. He told Albie this was a big adventure and to be brave. Dr. Nori told Albie he was a very brave little bear and she along with everyone at Neko Harbour Hospital were going to help him.

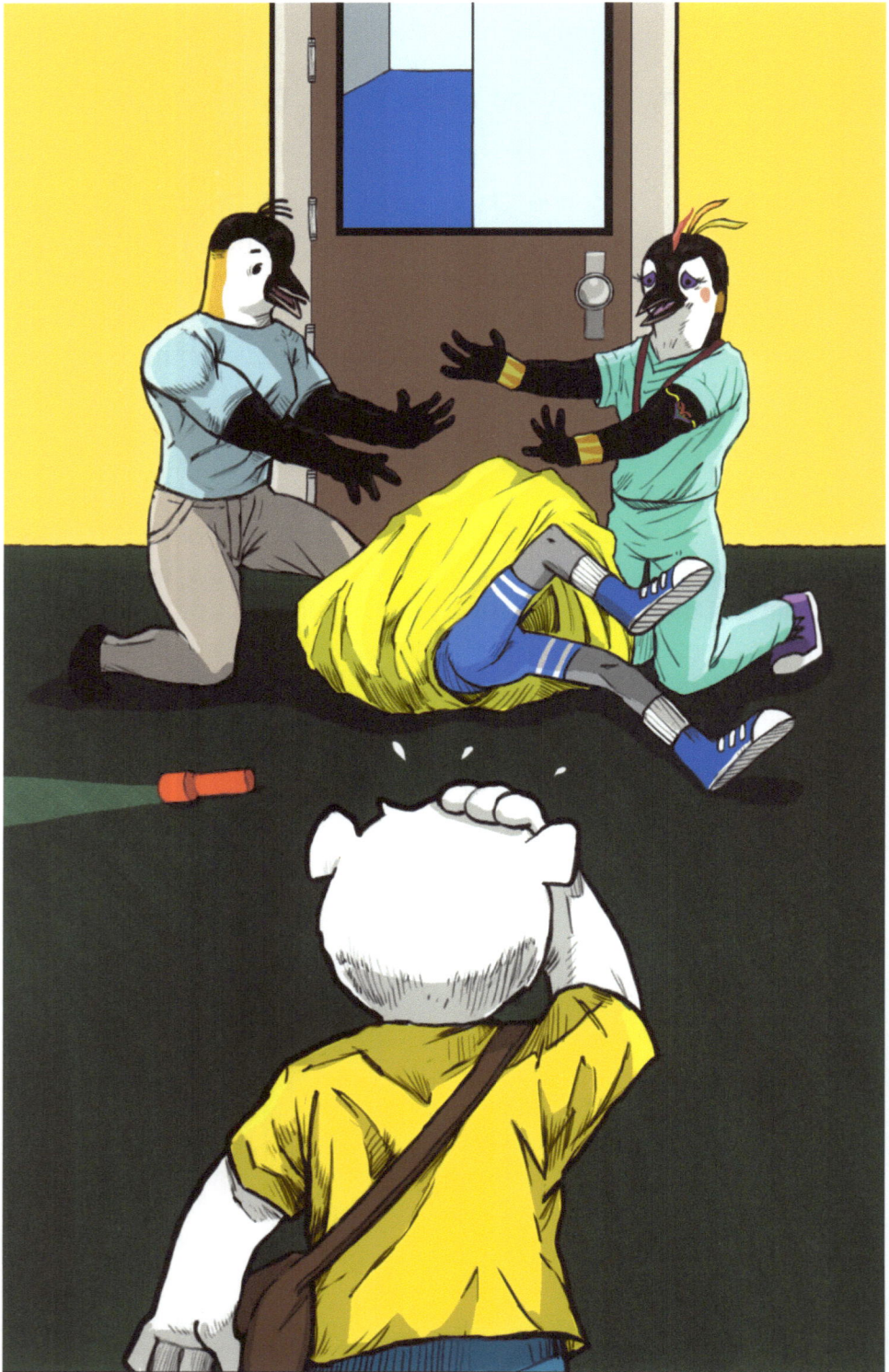

SUPER DANNY

Dr. Nori told Artemis to take Albie to his room and then he could have dinner with the other children. Albie got out his map and compass and followed Artemis. NORTH! Albie said, "We are going north." He was still thinking about Danny and wondering how he was doing. Albie thought to himself about what Tippy had said about how sometimes Danny sees things and hears things we don't. Tippy used that big word schizophrenia. Maybe that is what his mom and Dr. Nori meant by mental health. Albie hurt in his mind, but he didn't see or hear things like Danny. What was his mental illness then?

Albie noticed his compass starting to move. They were going east now. They were back in the long hallway with the windows. Albie could see all of Neko Harbour. He saw his Mom's hospital and the park. He could also see Mount Erebus, the great volcano on Ross Island. Albie saw his compass move once again and this time it was south. He started seeing pictures of Antarctica! They were awesome! There were pictures of Neko Harbour, Mount Erebus, Lake Vinson and wowwy, wow, The Great Ross Ice Shelf! Albie had always wanted to explore the ice shelves. He was paying so much attention to the pictures he didn't notice Artemis led him to his room. He heard a familiar voice and turned to see Tippy! She was rocking back and forth, plucking her feathers out nervously.

"Your room is right next door to mine!" Tippy told him. "My room has lots of books in it! I am going to be a psychiatrist like Dr. Nori one day. All my books are about psychology and the different medicines they use for mental illness. I got them from the library." Tippy was so excited. Albie thought she was very neat and told Tippy once more about him being an explorer and traveling all over the world. Tippy stopped plucking her feathers and asked to see his compass.

Tippy liked his compass. It was shiny and she liked how it showed her directions. Tippy held it as she began to spin real fast so the needle in the instrument would spin with her while she laughed out loud. Artemis asked Tippy to give the compass back so they could go to dinner. Albie hadn't even seen his room yet. Albie was told that he was sharing a room with Uni. He got so excited. Uni wants to be an explorer just like him. We are going to have so much fun together, he thought.

When Artemis opened the door to the room Albie was amazed! There was a glow in the dark globe that had light up flags all over the place. The room was dark, but there was enough light to see that Uni had all kinds of cool trinkets and collections of things. He had stuff that Albie wanted to know about. The curtains in the room were slightly closed, but the sun shined through and there was an aisle of light that stopped right in front of Albie's paws. Uni's side was by the door so Artemis led Albie to the bed by the window. He liked that his Mom and Dad had left him a bag and a letter which said how much they loved him.

There was something missing though? Artemis said Albie was sharing a room with Uni. Well, he couldn't see Uni anywhere. All his stuff was in the room but he wasn't there and he was with Tippy when Albie left the group. "Artemis? Where is Uni?"Albie asked. "Oh, he is in water therapy in the pool. It is very helpful to him and he loves to dive." "Therapy, what is therapy?" Albie asked. "Therapy helps give you understanding about your feelings and emotions," Artemis explained. "It gives you a way to find relief from stress. There are all different kinds of therapy" said Artemis. "Art therapy and music therapy are some of my favorites."

Albie wondered if he would have to do therapy and what type would he do. Just then there was a knock at the door, it was Danny! He had his blanket and two flashlights now. "I brought you something, Albie. Flashlights are good to see in the dark and you can make shadow puppets with them too." Albie was intrigued with Danny. He was just in the group and very upset, but now he was fine again. Albie thanked him for the flashlight and Danny twirled his blanket around. Before Albie could say anything else Danny ran back to his room.

Albie's tummy started to get hungry. He didn't want to get angry, but he was starting to growl a little. "Albie," Artemis said. "Are you okay?" Albie told her he needed something to eat. "I have just the place for us to go! Follow me," she said.

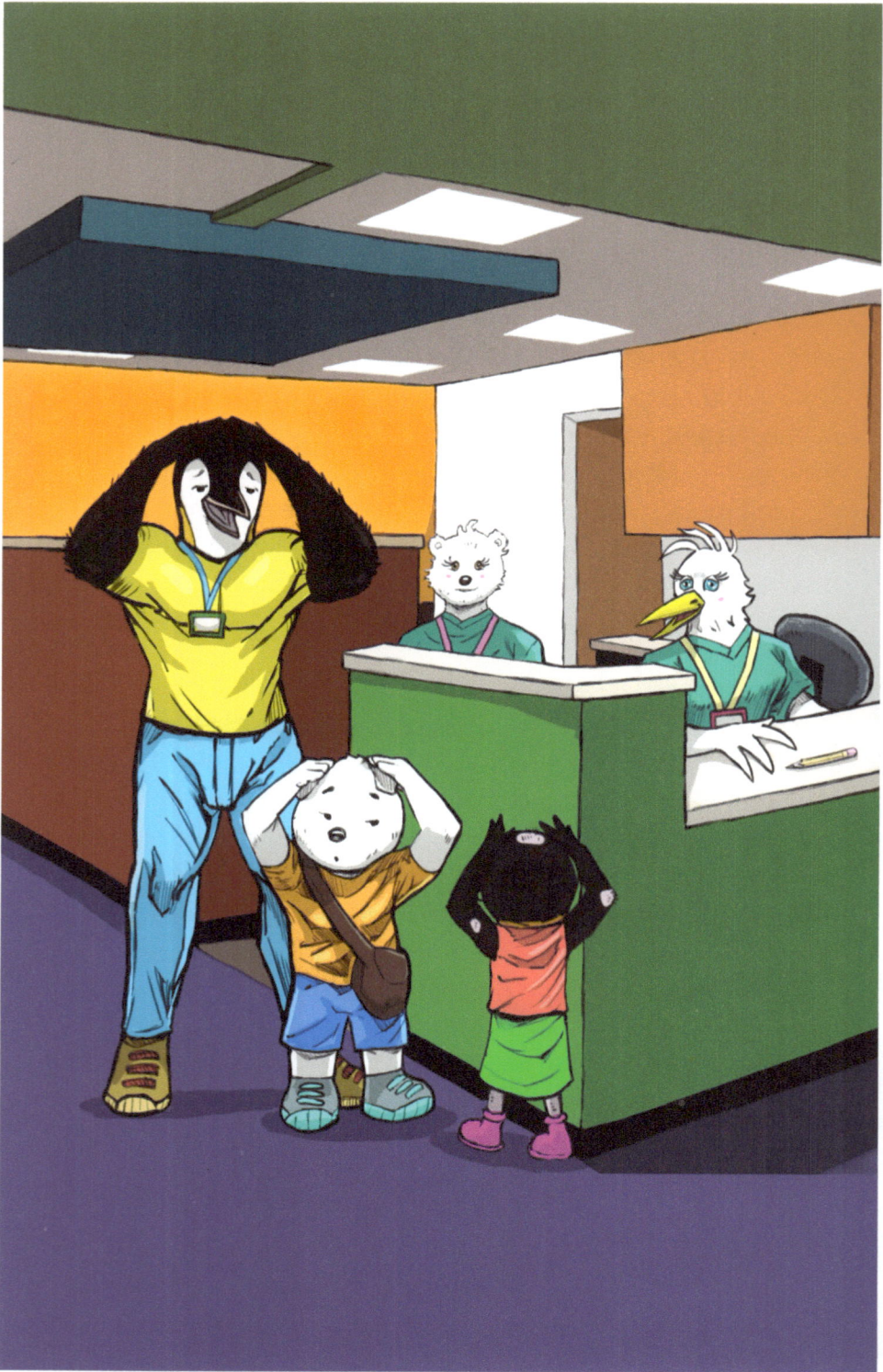

TAKING DEEP BREATHS WITH WALTER

Artemis led Albie to the Nurse's station right out front of the children's rooms. Walter was there and gave Albie a fist bump. "Walter, will you please make the dinner announcement so we can feed these hungry children." Walter called all the children to the Nurse's station. Albie was looking for Uni when all of a sudden he felt a tug on his fur. It was Tippy again and she was plucking her feathers! Excited, she said, "I just wanted to say hi again! We get to go eat now! "

Albie gave her a big smile as she had a book in her hands. It said all you need to know about anxiety. Albie thought I have never heard about anxiety before. "Tippy, what is anxiety?"Albie asked. "Well, I think it's when I get nervous or scared sometimes about something and I pluck my feathers. Dr.Nori gave me medicine to take and I go to therapy that helps me. Walter gave me this book too." "That was very nice of them to help you," Albie said. Albie was hoping they could help him too. Medicine and therapy for what though?

Albie still did not know what his mental illness was. He didn't get anxiety that he knew of and he wasn't like Danny. He didn't see things that weren't there. What about Uni he thought, did Uni take medicine? Albie had so many questions, but his tummy was hungry .He couldn't stand it. He couldn't help it. He couldn't stop it. All of a sudden he let out a loud GROWL!!!! Tippy covered her ears and crouched down. Danny covered his head with his blanket. Uni's jaw dropped in fear of what was wrong with his new friend.

Walter quickly came to Albie's rescue and tried to get him to breathe. "Lift your paws young cub. Inhale when you lift and exhale when you bring them down. Everyone else did the breathing with Albie and Walter. Albie soon calmed down and Artemis asked him if he would get his compass out so she could show him where the cafeteria was. Albie thanked her and hugged Walter for his help in calming him down. "Just don't forget to breathe Albie. It always helps me."

The cafeteria was on the west side of the hospital according to Albie's map and compass. Danny had his flashlight on while Tippy and Uni were still practicing breathing. Albie began to smell the air. Oh my, his tummy was hungry. He could smell the fresh fish and sushi. He was going to eat so much. When he turned the corner to enter the cafeteria Albie saw Dr. Nori. She had a big plate of silver fish. Dr. Nori waved and smiled real big at all of the children. Danny shined his flashlight on her and then scooted real fast to get his dinner. Tippy shouted "Hello" as she jumped up and down waving! Tippy had a lot of energy, Albie thought to himself. Albie wondered where Uni went. He had just seen him with Tippy. Uni called to Albie from behind him. "Albie, do you like sushi?" Uni had two huge plates of fresh sushi and Albie's eyes popped wide open! They all went to sit down. Tippy and Danny were sitting by Artemis. Walter was on the other side of the table.

Walter was the biggest penguin Albie had ever seen. He was very smart too. He had helped Albie to breathe when he got mad and growled. Uni plopped down right by Walter and Albie sat next to Uni. Albie apologized for growling and scaring everyone. Walter said, "It's not necessary to apologize. Everyone has their own way of expressing their emotions." Albie thought for a moment about that word, emotions? He asked Walter what he meant by that. What are emotions? Walter explained that Albie's anger was an emotion or feeling that he had. Walter told Albie there are all different sorts of emotions; sad, happy, angry and even scared. Everyone has emotions and feelings. It's how we react to them that sometimes make us different. Walter told Albie that he liked to lift weights. If he got mad he would lift weights. If he got sad he would lift weights and even when he was happy, he lifted weights. Walter said, "If I can't lift weights, I just practice breathing with my emotions. I like to talk about my emotions," said Danny. When I get scared, I say "Fear, I will shine my light on you and you will be bright so I can see you!" Albie and the others laughed at Danny. "There are many ways to handle your emotions and feelings. This is what makes us all unique and wonderful individuals." Everyone turned around to see Dr. Nori as she spoke. She was so majestic!

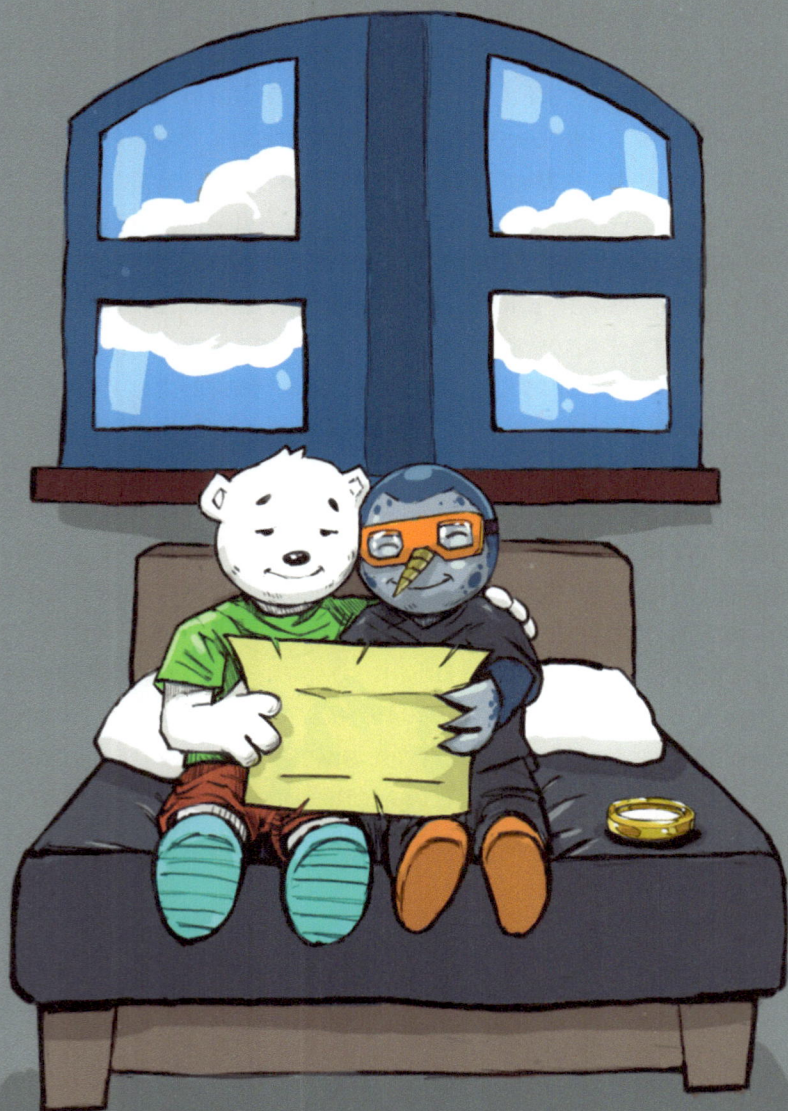

DEPRESSION AND AN
UNDERSTANDING FRIEND

Dr. Nori asked Albie to come with her so she could speak with him. Albie thought he might be in trouble for growling, but that wasn't the case at all. She wanted to start Albie's tests so they could find what his diagnosis and treatment were going to be. Dr. Nori explained she was going to take Albie to get a brain scan so she can see anything to help her with Albie's diagnosis. Albie wondered what a brain scan was. He started to get a little nervous. How was she going to scan his brain? Did she have to cut his head open to take his brain out? Was he going to bleed? Albie's mind was all over the place with questions. He grabbed his satchel tight and followed Dr. Nori to a room with a large machine in it. Albie said, "Are you going to take my brain out?" Dr. Nori laughed, "No Albie, I'm going to take pictures of your brain with this machine. This is called a Magnetic Resonance Imaging (MRI) machine. It's like a big camera that can see inside your body." "Wow!" Albie said. "I thought this was going to be scary for a minute!" Albie put his satchel with his map and compass down before he laid down on the large machine. Dr. Nori turned on some soft music for him, turned off the lights and told Albie to look at the stars above his head. Albie looked above his head at the stars, listened to the music and let the machine scan his brain. When Albie was done with the MRI he was exhausted. He had done so much today meeting many new children and adults. He had learned so much about mental health, but he still didn't know what was wrong with him. Why was he here? It was still bugging him. He was frustrated and tired. Dr. Nori took Albie back to his room. Albie saw Uni was asleep in his bed already. Dr. Nori told Albie he could call his Mom and Dad if he wanted or he could wait until the morning. Albie wanted to call, but he just wanted to sleep. He took off his satchel, put his pajamas on and snuggled up in his bed.

Albie was sound asleep when he started hearing whimpering and crying on Uni's side of the room. Albie couldn't tell what was happening. It was too dark. "Uni," Albie called. "Is that you?" Albie got his flashlight and turned it toward Uni's side of the room. Uni was curled up in a ball with his pillow over his head. "Uni, what are you doing over there? Are you upset?" Uni quietly said, "I have nobody. My parents are gone. Nobody wants me and I will be here forever." Albie didn't know what to do. He was sad his friend was feeling so bad. He tried to pat Uni on the back, but Uni still sobbed. Then Albie remembered something Walter said about emotions. Uni was having sad emotions right now. Albie told Uni to try and breathe, that Albie was there for him and Uni would be okay. Albie went to his satchel and got out a map he had of the world. He took it back to Uni and told him to look at it. Uni sat up and looked at the map. Albie told him all the places he wanted to go and asked Uni to show him on the map where he had been. Uni pointed to the Arctic Ocean and said it was the last place he saw his family. Albie told Uni since he was going to be a great explorer he would help Uni find his family one day. Uni smiled and said, "I will explore with you Albie!" The two friends snuggled up next to each other falling asleep with the map and flashlight still on.

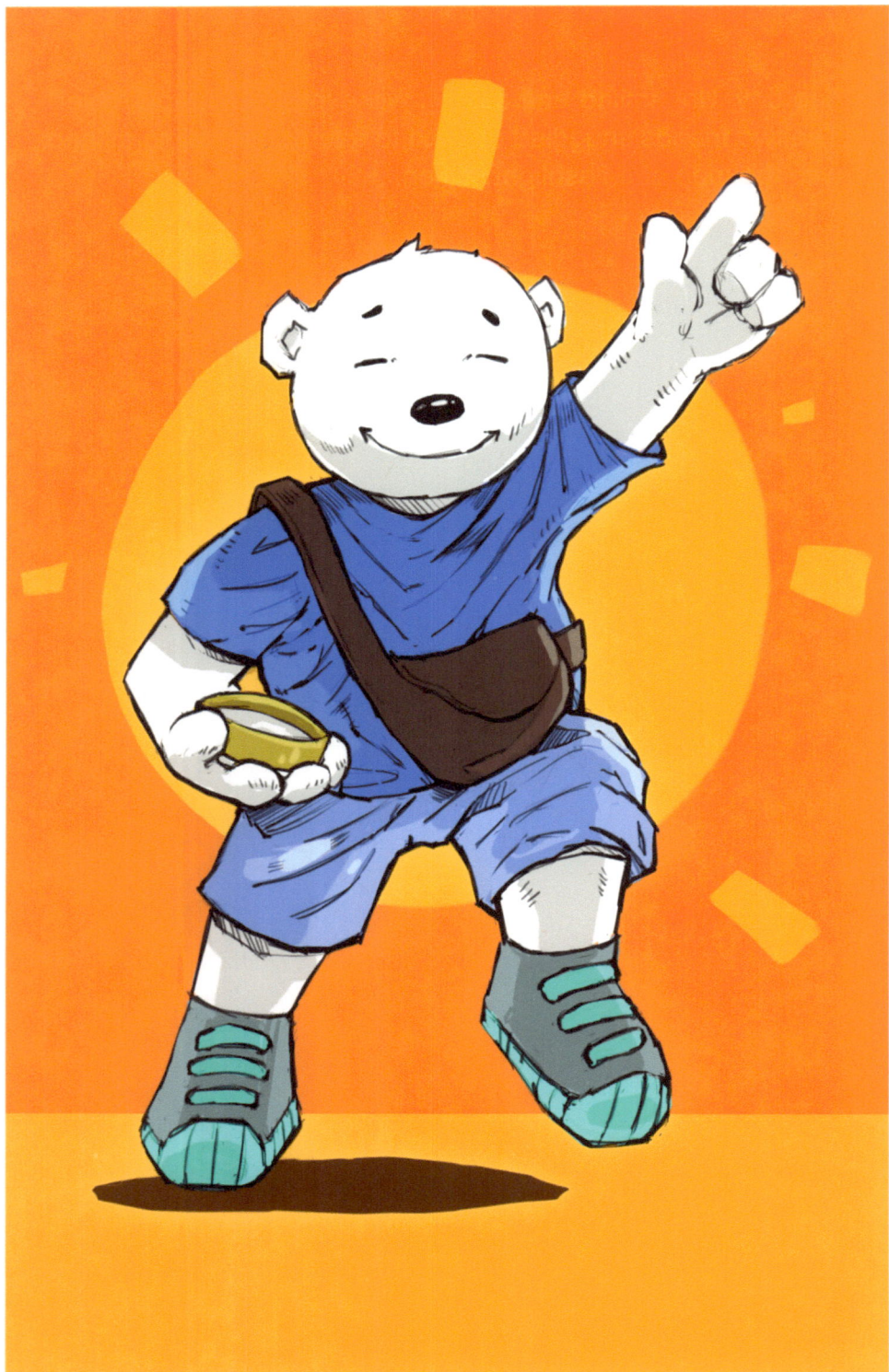

A DIAGNOSIS

Albie woke up to Artemis singing and dancing in their room. Uni was still asleep. Albie wanted to call his Mom and Dad. He wanted them to know about his new friends. He wanted to tell them about his brain scan. He wanted them to know about the cafeteria and how all the food was so delicious. When he called he also told them how he lost his temper again and how Uni cried in the night. His Mom and Dad told Albie how brave he had been and they were sure he would be able to come home soon.

Albie was feeling really happy and excited. What was he going to do today? Artemis called Albie and told him to meet Walter in the art room. Albie got his map out and his compass then went about his way. Albie saw Walter sitting at the table with a set of paints and colors. Walter gave his big ole high five to Albie then asked him to sit down with him. Walter explained, "This is the room in the hospital where we do art therapy, Albie. You can paint, color or draw and it helps us with your diagnosis." It all sounded good to Albie. Walter pulled out a folder that had blank sheets of paper inside. Walter told Albie to use paints or colors to draw whatever he wanted. Albie thought for a minute then started with a picture of Mount Erebus. The more he drew the more he remembered what he had done to come to the hospital in the first place. He knew the answer and didn't get picked. Shayla got picked to answer. Albie began to get angry again thinking about that day. He started to get upset and cry. He didn't want to get mad today, but couldn't control himself. Walter tapped Albie on his shoulder and said, "Remember Albie, just breathe, you are okay. You are safe and I am here for you." Walter gave Albie his picture and Albie told Walter what had happened. Walter told Albie about coping skills. These were ways to help Albie deal with his anger and sadness as well as other emotions. Walter reminded Albie about breathing and trying to think a happy thought like exploring or to picture in your mind something you like. Albie thought hard about what Walter was saying. Albie asked to color and draw another picture. This picture was going to be one of all his new friends at Neko Harbour Hospital.

Albie helped Walter clean up the paint and color. Walter was showing Albie some other pictures when they heard a knock at the door. Albie turned around and saw his Mom and Dad! He ran over to them as fast as he could and hugged them both tightly. Oh, he was so happy to see them! "Look at what I drew!" he said, showing his parents the pictures of Mount Erebus and his new friends. Walter and Albie's parents said hello to each other. Albie told his Mom and Dad that Walter was a therapist who taught Albie some coping skills for his anger and sadness. Albie's Dad told them he had to learn coping skills when he was in the military. Walter and Albie's Dad started talking as Albie's Mom told that Dr. Nori had asked them to come to the hospital. "We are supposed to have a visit with her now." Albie was a little nervous, but very curious to find out what Dr. Nori had to say. Was it going to be about his diagnosis maybe?

Walter took Albie and his parents to see Dr. Nori. It was such a long walk for Albie. What was she going to say to them? Was he going to have to take another test or did she finally know what was wrong with him? His mind wouldn't stop. Albie's Mom grabbed his paw and smiled. "All will be okay, Albie. Just continue to be brave and all will be fine." Oh, how Albie loved his Mom. She always knew how to make him feel better. They got to Dr. Nori's office and she was standing beside a computer screen with two pictures on it. They looked funny to Albie. He couldn't tell what they were, but there were different colors on both pictures in certain spots. "Oh, hello," said Dr. Nori. "Come in, come in. It's so good to see you." She asked Albie how art therapy went with Walter so Albie showed her the pictures he drew. Dr. Nori was in one of the pictures. She loved them both. Albie was happy to see Dr. Nori, but he wanted to know what those pictures were on the computer screen. He was so curious he couldn't think of anything else. Walter said goodbye and told Albie what a good job he did in therapy. He told Albie's parents it was nice to meet them.

Dr. Nori asked Albie and his parents to sit down so she could talk with them about Albie's diagnosis. Diagnosis, Albie thought? She knows what's wrong with me. She asked them if they had ever heard of Bipolar Disorder. Bipolar disorder, Albie wondered? What is that! Albie's parents looked at each other and said "Yes." Colonel Polar Bear had a friend in the Arctic Army with Bipolar and Albie's Mom had seen it from her experience as a nurse. Albie thought okay, okay, everyone knows this, but what about me? I don't know this Bipolar! Albie started to get upset because he didn't understand.

Dr. Nori looked over at Albie and asked him to come over to her side of the desk. Albie walked over and she showed him the big computer screen. Dr. Nori said, "Albie, these are pictures of your brain from the MRI we took." Albie looked at the picture. There were red, yellow, green and blue colors all over his brain. There were two sides in the picture, the right side of his brain and the left. The coloring on Albie's brain was lighter and darker in some areas and there was more of a certain color in others. Then Dr. Nori showed them another picture of a brain and said it was called a control brain that belonged to someone else. Dr. Nori said, "Albie's picture shows signs of Bipolar Disorder. The other picture is a brain without."

Albie started to get upset again. "What is Bipolar?" Albie said. "Everyone knows but me and I am the one you're talking about." Dr. Nori smiled at Albie and looked at his parents. "I am sorry. I didn't mean to upset you. Bipolar Disorder is when you have episodes of mood swings where you can be really happy one minute and really sad or mad another. It is a mental illness. The MRI is just a tool to help me see a part of your diagnosis. Counselor Prion and you telling me stories of your behaviors and emotions helped me come to my diagnosis as well."

Dr. Nori told them with medication and therapy they could treat Albie. Therapy and medicine Albie thought? Albie's Mom and Dad continued to talk to Dr. Nori. All Albie could do was think about Bipolar. That's what his mental illness was! That's why he gets so upset and can't control his anger and sadness. He's Bipolar! I am a Bipolar Bear, Albie thought. He finally had an answer to his questions. Albie kept thinking about it and what it was going to be like taking medicine and going to therapy. He liked art therapy with Walter, but medicine? What was that going to be like?

Dr. Nori told Albie and his parents she wanted to start Albie on some medicine for his Bipolar illness. She wanted him to stay a little longer at the hospital so they can watch over him to see how he reacts to the medicine. Albie was excited to tell his new friends about what happened today. He wanted to tell them he was now on medicine and knew what was causing his problems. It was Bipolar. Albie's parents asked him if he needed anything and he said no. They told Albie they would talk to him later in the evening after dinner. Albie was going to miss them, but he knew his diagnosis now. He couldn't wait to share that with everyone. He jumped up. His Mom and Dad came in for a group hug. "We are proud of you kiddo! You have been so brave."